# Health Technical Memorandum 2040

Validation and verification

## The control of legionellae in healthcare premises – a code of practice

London: HMSO

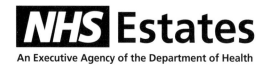

An Executive Agency of the Department of Health

ISBN 0 11 321681 5

*Cover photograph:*
Scanning electron micrograph of a biofilm on latex showing
amoeba grazing the bacterial consortium (magnification x 1440).
Reproduced by kind permission of Julie Rogers and A B Dowsett,
Public Health Laboratory Service Centre for Applied Microbiology
and Research, Porton Down, Salisbury, Wiltshire.

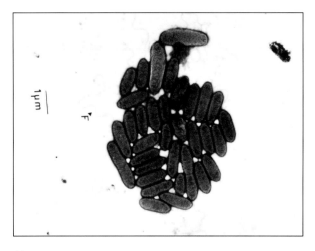

*Above:*
A colony of bacteria *Legionella pneumophila.* The bacteria are
non-sporing, typically 2–3 μm long, 0.3–0.9 μm wide. Flagella,
which can be clearly seen, provide mobility of the organism.
Reproduced by kind permission of Public Health Laboratory
Service Centre for Applied Microbiology and Research.

**HMSO**
**Standing order service**

Placing a standing order with HMSO BOOKS enables a
customer to receive future titles in this series automatically
as published. This saves the time, trouble and expense of
placing individual orders and avoids the problem of
knowing when to do so. For details please write to HMSO
BOOKS (PC 13A/1), Publications Centre, PO Box 276,
London SW8 5DT quoting reference 14 02 017.
The standing order service also enables customers to receive
automatically as published all material of their choice which
additionally saves extensive catalogue research. The scope
and selectivity of the service has been extended by new
techniques, and there are more than 3,500 classifications to
choose from. A special leaflet describing the service in detail
may be obtained on request.

# About this publication

Health Technical Memorandum (HTM) 2040 provides recommendations, advice and guidance on controlling legionellae in healthcare premises. It is applicable to new and existing sites, and is for use at various stages during the inception, design, upgrading, refurbishment, extension and maintenance of a building.

HTM 2040 focuses on the:

   a. legal and mandatory requirements;

   b. design of systems;

   c. maintenance of systems;

   d. operation of systems.

It is published as five separate volumes, each addressing a specialist discipline:

   a. **Management policy** – outlines the overall responsibility of managers of healthcare premises, and details their legal and mandatory obligations. It summarises the essential background information required to understand the principles of the control of legionellae. This is followed by an epidemiology of legionellosis, essential to understanding the rationale behind the various control and design measures advocated in succeeding volumes;

   b. **Design considerations** – highlights the overall requirements and considerations that should be applied to the design up to the contract document;

   c. this volume – **Validation and verification** – considers the testing and commissioning aspects, also providing guidance on the identification of problem areas;

   d. **Operational management** – considers aspects of preventing and controlling legionellae. It also contains information on the operation, maintenance and cleaning of evaporative cooling towers;

   e. **Good practice guide** – gives advice on the course of action if an outbreak of legionnaires' disease is suspected, on the cleaning and disinfection of a cooling tower implicated in an outbreak of legionnaires' disease, and on the use of sodium hypochlorite solutions for chlorination of cooling water systems in hospitals. Further advice is given in the form of:

(i) emptying times for cooling tower ponds;

(ii) a questionnaire to assess the serviceability of existing cooling systems;

(iii) a sample logbook for the planned maintenance of a cooling tower.

Guidance in this Health Technical Memorandum is complemented by the library of National Health Service Model Engineering Specifications. Users of the guidance are advised to refer to the relevant specifications.

The contents of this Health Technical Memorandum in terms of management policy, operational policy and technical guidance are endorsed by:

a. the Welsh Office for the NHS in Wales;

b. the Health and Personal Social Services Management Executive in Northern Ireland;

c. the National Health Service in Scotland Management Executive;

and they set standards consistent with Departmental Cost Allowances.

This HTM was written with the advice and assistance of experts in the NHS and industry.

References to legislation appearing in the main text of this guidance apply in England and Wales. Where references differ for Scotland and/or Northern Ireland these are given in marginal notes.

Where appropriate, marginal notes are also used to amplify the text.

# Contents

# 1.0 Introduction

**1.1** The guidance contained in this volume is applicable to new and existing sites, and is for use at various stages during the inception, design, upgrading, refurbishment, extensions and maintenance of a building.

**1.2** The approach should be to remove all potential sources of seeding, growth and spread of legionellae. Where this ideal cannot be achieved in existing situations, steps should be taken to control and prevent legionellae by sound operational management.

**1.3** The control of legionellae is a continuing responsibility. Effectiveness of precautionary measures should be continually monitored, and a continuing programme to ensure awareness should be devised. Although knowledge of legionellosis has improved markedly in recent years, there is a continuing misunderstanding about the method of dissemination. Many people are under the impression that cooling towers are the only source of legionellae in building service systems. All water systems are capable of colonisation by legionellae, and taps are just as capable of generating an aerosol as showers or indeed cooling towers.

**1.4** The biggest risk is complacency, leading to the deterioration of water hygiene to the extent that an outbreak of the disease occurs.

**1.5** Good practice design alone will not prevent outbreaks of legionellae.

**1.6** The HTM does not include advice on water supplies for clinical equipment such as dialysers, nebulisers and respiratory humidifiers, nor for sterile water services for pharmacy departments. Users of clinical humidifiers and nebulisers are reminded that sterile water, not tap water, should be used and that they should be emptied and cleaned thoroughly following each period of use. All equipment with water reservoirs should be stored dry. Water for any purpose should meet functional and local requirements, but users must recognise that any water system may provide a suitable environment for legionellae and other water-borne organisms and systems should therefore be designed to take account of this.

# 2.0 Validation and verification considerations

## Commissioning and testing of hot and cold water systems

**2.1**   The hot and cold water service systems should be commissioned and tested in accordance with BS6700 and HTM 27 – 'Cold water supply storage and mains distribution'. BS6700 details procedures to ensure that:

    a. materials and equipment installed comply with other British Standards and are not otherwise unsuitable;

    b. the work is done entirely within the specification for the scheme;

    c. the installation complies in every respect with current water byelaws and regulations and the requirements of British Standards;

    d. all the requirements of current legislation are met, both during construction of the installation and when it is completed, particularly with regard to the Health and Safety at Work etc Act 1974.

*Northern Ireland: Health and Safety at Work (NI) Order 1978*

*Scotland: SOHHD PIL/8/9*

**2.2**   "As installed" drawings and operating/maintenance instructions must be supplied at the time of handover. Schematics will also be useful. Certified records of pressure testing and disinfection should also be made available.

*See SHHD/DGM (1990)80 – Hot and Cold Water Services*

## Pressure testing

**2.3**   Pressure testing must be carried out before disinfection. Except where otherwise specified, testing of underground pipelines should be carried out in accordance with BS5886, CP312 and CP2010, as appropriate for the pipeline material.

**2.4**   Open pipes should be capped and valves closed to avoid contamination. After pressure testing it will be impracticable to drain the system completely.

## Disinfection

**2.5**   The system should be disinfected in accordance with BS6700. Disinfection should be carried out within seven days of the system being brought into use unless:

    a. hot water temperatures are maintained;

    b. cold water temperatures are maintained;

    c. regular (every seven days) flushing is carried out.

*The contract should specify this for the period that the system is under the contractor's control*

*Scotland: Refer to SHTN No 2 for detail*

**2.6**   Once filled, systems should not be drained unless full disinfection is to be undertaken before the system is brought into use again.

**2.7**   For design and build contracts, the brief must include the requirement that adequate certification of disinfection is provided by the contractor. On other contracts, tests must be witnessed and certified. During the post-handover period prior to occupation it is the client's responsibility to ensure system temperatures are maintained and regular flushing is carried out, or to implement full re-disinfection.

## Temperature testing

**2.8**   These tests should be performed prior to contractural handover and bringing the system into use. Separate thermometric measuring and recording equipment should be used, that is, independent of any building management system. It will be necessary to have systems fully operational and to simulate typical draw-off of water.

**2.9**   Tests should include:

a.  measuring the incoming water temperature at the water meter;

b.  testing the inlet, outlet and surface water temperatures of cisterns and cold water feed/header tanks for the hot water calorifiers. The temperature should not be greater than 2°C above that measured at (a);

c.  testing the flow and return temperatures of calorifiers and boilers. These should not be less than 60°C and 50°C respectively;

d.  testing the temperature at hot and cold water draw-off points, at sinks, wash-hand basins and baths, etc. A steady state temperature of between 50°C and 60°C at hot water draw-off should be reached within one minute. At cold water draw-off a temperature of not greater than 2°C above the temperature measured at (a) should be reached within one minute.

## Discharge of waste water used during disinfection procedures within buildings

*Northern Ireland: Health and Safety Agency for Northern Ireland Publication HSA 62*

**2.10**   External bodies responsible for sewers should be informed before chlorinated water used for disinfecting an installation is discharged. Additional disinfection guidance is given in HS(G)70. It is preferable, therefore, to establish and agree procedures beforehand; this may simply involve the dilution of the discharge or de-chlorination.

**2.11**   When required, de-chlorination can be achieved using either sulphur dioxide or sodium thiosulphate (20 g of sodium thiosulphate crystals is required to de-chlorinate 500 litres of water containing 20 mg/l free chlorine).

**2.12**   If possible, it may be preferable to add the sodium thiosulphate to the chlorinated water at the point of discharge into the foul sewer rather than into systems. This will avoid the need for draining and washing systems of any residual chemical which would otherwise mop up any chlorine that may be present in the water.

# 3.0 Cold water systems

## General

**3.1**  The requirements for disinfection subsequent to flushing out to remove debris, etc are essentially those given in BS6700. Further guidance is available in 'A Guide to Pre-Commission Cleaning of Water Systems', issued by BSRIA, 1991, which deals with the design/installation considerations, system flushing and chemical cleaning. Background notes on disinfection by chlorine are given in HTM 2040, 'Good practice guide', Appendix 1.

**3.2**  Alternative disinfectants may be used provided satisfactory disinfection is achieved. The infection control team should be consulted.

**3.3**  Proprietary solutions of disinfectant should be used in accordance with the manufacturers' instructions and will have to take due regard of the requirements under COSHH and other health and safety regulations.

**3.4**  A suitable proprietary test kit should be used for site measurements of residual disinfection agents.

**3.5**  Disinfection should not be undertaken before materials, for example linings in cisterns, have fully cured.

## Installations outside buildings

**3.6**  Pipework under pressure from the mains should be disinfected through an injection point and the disinfectant residual measured at the end of the pipeline. It is normal water industry practice to use a chlorine dose of not less than 20 mg/l (ppm) and, because the nature of the installation is likely to lead to unavoidable contamination, it is usual practice to leave the chlorine solution in the pipes for 24 hours before thoroughly flushing out with fresh water. Junctions which are to be inserted into existing pipelines should be disinfected prior to installation.

**3.7**  All disinfection of pipework under pressure from the mains must be carried out in accordance with the requirements of the local water undertaking. Failure to ensure close liaison between the contractor and the water authority during design, construction, pressure testing or commissioning could present a potential risk of back-siphonage of contaminated materials or chemicals into the public water supply. Site supervision to ensure compliance with any requirements specified by the local water authority is strongly recommended.

## Cold water installations within buildings

**3.8**  All cistern(s) should be internally cleaned to remove all visible dirt and debris. Cistern(s) and distributing pipework should be drained, filled with fresh water and then drained completely. The cistern(s) should then be refilled and their supply servicing valves closed. On re-fitting it is normal practice to add high doses of sodium hypochlorite to the water in the cistern(s), for example to give a calculated chlorine concentration of 50 ± 10 mg/l (ppm) in the water and leave the water to stand for one hour. Whatever disinfection method is used, the concentration should be adjusted if necessary. The use of a high dose ensures an adequate residual concentration to allow proper disinfection of the downstream services. Each tap or fitting should then be opened, progressively away from the cistern(s), and water discharged until the disinfectant is detected. Each tap or fitting should then be closed, and the cistern and pipes left charged for a further one hour. The tap(s) furthest from the cistern(s) should be opened and the level of disinfectant in the water discharged from the tap(s) measured. If the levels set in the British Standards are not achieved the disinfection process should be repeated.

**3.9**   As soon as possible after disinfection, the distribution pipework should be drained and thoroughly flushed through with fresh water and re-filled. Appropriate hazard warnings should be placed on the taps throughout the building during disinfection procedures.

**3.10**   After disinfection, microbiological tests for bacterial colony counts at 22°C and 37°C and coliform bacteria including *Escherichia coli* for drinking water should be carried out under the supervision of the infection control team to establish that the work has been satisfactorily completed. Water samples should be taken from selected areas within the distribution system. The system should not be brought into service until the infection control team certifies that the water is of potable quality.

## Storage cisterns

**3.11**   Cold water storage cisterns are installed in the majority of hospital buildings/departments. A maximum of 24 hours' total on-site storage capacity is recommended. The quantity of water stored should be carefully assessed in relation to the daily requirement in order that a reasonable rate of turnover is achieved. Storage of unnecessarily large quantities of potable water will result in low rates of turnover and a consequent deterioration in the quality of water. The storage capacity should be reduced where it is known or established that it is excessive and where it is practicable to do so. An example would be where there are two cisterns in parallel, one of which can be left empty and blanked-off (pipe sections should be removed). Alternatively, the steady water level in the cisterns should be lowered. This can be done most easily if the float controlling the water supply has a thumbscrew adjustment as prescribed in BS1212: Part 2. The design capacity should not allow for future extensions.

# 4.0 Hot water services

## Hot water installations within buildings

**4.1**    Cold feed cisterns, hot water calorifiers, water heaters, direct-fired HWS boilers and distribution pipework should be disinfected in accordance with paragraphs 3.8 to 3.11; no heat source should be applied during the disinfection procedure, including final flushing.

# 5.0 Evaporative cooling towers

## General

**5.1**   The following paragraphs give general guidance on the operation and maintenance of cooling towers.

**5.2**   Before the identification of legionellae and its association with evaporative cooling systems, cooling towers were maintained for maximum service life. The aim of maintenance was to minimise fouling, thus ensuring optimum thermal efficiency.

**5.3**   Most evaporative cooling systems are uncomplicated in construction, simple in operation and usually located close to the refrigeration plant. Significant deterioration is possible, therefore, before plant inefficiency becomes evident.

**5.4**   It is essential that the utmost care and diligence is exercised in the operation and maintenance of cooling towers. The operation, maintenance and water treatment of evaporative cooling systems must be considered with regard to the associated health risks, in addition to operational efficiency.

## Operating and maintenance documents

**5.5**   Operating and maintenance documents must be available for each installation and must be complete at the time of handover. If unavailable, operating and maintenance documents must be prepared by the user and should include the following:

- a. the design intent description, usually prepared by the designer and including the system function and its description. It should also include the design requirements in respect of water treatment regimen, flow rates, static and dynamic pressures, thermal capacities, system volumes, operating temperatures, control sensor locations, operating set points and all other relevant information. If commissioning information is not available it will be necessary to recommission the plant in order to prepare records of the operational parameters of the entire system;

- b. a description of how the plant and system as a whole are set to work and how they are shut down;

- c. a fault diagnosis schedule, description of the alarm/warning system and details of courses of corrective/diagnostic action in event of a fault condition. The schedule should also include a checklist and give guidance on checking possible causes of complaint originating from the occupier;

- d. manufacturer's installation instructions and literature;

- e. spares information;

- f. operation instructions for individual items of plant;

- g. maintenance information for individual items of plant and maintenance frequencies;

- h. record drawings of the installation;

*Schedule 3 of the Consumer Protection Act 1987 required that sufficient information is made available to the operator for him/her to safely operate the plant*

J.  plantroom and system schematic diagrams (framed copies should be mounted in the respective plantrooms);

k.  lubrication charts with frequencies;

m.  valve charts showing valve number, type and purpose and, where applicable, design flows/settings/pressure drops;

n.  logbooks.

## Logbooks

**5.6**  The purpose of a logbook system is to improve the efficiency and effectiveness of installation and maintenance, and also to provide a record of various tasks and observations so that the plant history can be reviewed at any time by the maintenance engineer. It will prove essential to the maintenance engineer in the operation of a planned plant maintenance scheme, and, if properly followed, will prevent unacceptable conditions developing as a result of ineffective maintenance.

**5.7**  The logbook should:

a.  identify the installation requiring attention, in this case an evaporative cooling system, and should describe its form, function and how it operates;

b.  record the results of the initial commissioning and any recommissioning so that observations made during maintenance checks can be compared;

c.  define the maintenance task or observation required and the frequency;

d.  provide for the recording of maintenance observations and results and for comments to be made in respect of any defect seen during the inspection. This facility should exist for each item of plant individually and for overall system observations;

e.  provide preliminary guidance on fault diagnosis and checking to assist with immediate on-site correction or adjustment;

f.  provide for, and make reference to, any separate observation sheet required to record extensive or abnormal observations which cannot be noted on the routine inspection sheets;

g.  facilitate cataloguing and cross-referencing to other logbooks for plant/installations on the same site (for example, the refrigeration plant, the chilled water installation, the air-conditioning plant and the heat source).

*As an aid to the preparation of a suitable logbook system, a sample logbook for an evaporative cooling system is included in HTM 2040 'Good practice guide'*

## Operational checks

**5.8**  This section of the HTM is intended to assist maintenance staff in the planning of operational and functional checks. It identifies typical tasks and recommends observation frequencies. It is only a general guide, as it is not possible to cover all aspects which relate to a specific installation.

**5.9**  Details of operational and functional tasks must be drawn up for each site by the "nominated person". These, together with the completion of log sheets, will enable a proper historical record to be compiled of all works carried out and observations made.

**5.10**  Frequencies are indicated for initial guidance only, as they will vary to suit a particular site, its location, the design parameters and particular provisions, for example manual operation rather than automatic control methods.

**5.11**  The user's needs must be considered before commencing any operational or maintenance tasks. Where standby or dual facilities are not provided, the timing of these tasks must be carefully planned to minimise inconvenience.

# 6.0 Air-conditioning and mechanical ventilation

## General

**6.1**  Air-conditioning and ventilation plant and ductwork should be inspected at the access point(s) quarterly to see that it is clean and to report on its general condition.

## Fresh air inlet

**6.2**  In the case of existing installations the use of portable smoke generators or smoke bombs may be helpful in observing the discharge plume from cooling towers and discharges from extract systems in order to assess any potential risk.

*The wind conditions will vary from day to day and sufficient tests to provide a representative sample will be necessary. The tests should be repeated with the cooling tower fan(s) both on and off*

# Other publications in this series

(Given below are details of all Health Technical Memoranda available from HMSO. HTMs marked (*) are currently being revised, those marked (†) are out of print. Some HTMs in preparation at the time of publication of this HTM are also listed.)

  1  Anti-static precautions: rubber, plastics and fabrics*†

  2  Anti-static precautions: flooring in anaesthetising areas (and data processing rooms)*, 1977.

  3  –

  4  –

  5  Steam boiler plant instrumentation†

  6  Protection of condensate systems: filming amines†

2007  Electrical services: supply and distribution, 1993.

  8  –

  9  –

 10  Sterilizers*†

2011  Emergency electrical services, 1993.

 12  –

 13  –

2014  Abatement of electrical interference, 1993.

 15  Patient/nurse call systems†

 16  –

 17  Health building engineering installations: commissioning and associated activities, 1978.

 18  Facsimile telegraphy: possible applications in DGHs†

 19  Facsimile telegraphy: the transmission of pathology reports within a hospital – a case study†

2020  Electrical safety code for low voltage systems, 1993.

2021  Electrical safety code for high voltage systems, 1993.

 22  Piped medical gases, medical compressed air and medical vacuum installations*†

 22  Supp. Permit to work system: for piped medical gases etc†

 23  Access and accommodation for engineering services†

 24  –

 25  –

 26  Commissioning of oil, gas and dual fired boilers: with notes on design, operation and maintenance†

 27  Cold water supply storage and mains distribution* [Revised version will deal with water storage and distribution], 1978.

28 to 39 –

41 to 53 –

## Component Data Base (HTMs 54 to 70)

54.1 User manual, 1993.

55   Windows, 1989.

56   Partitions, 1989.

57   Internal glazing, 1989.

58   Internal doorsets, 1989.

59   Ironmongery, 1989.

60   Ceilings, 1989.

61   Flooring, 1989.

62   Demountable storage systems, 1989.

63   Fitted storage systems, 1989.

64   Sanitary assemblies, 1989.

65   Signs†

66   Cubicle curtain track, 1989.

67   Laboratory fitting-out system, 1993.

68   Ducts and panel assemblies, 1993.

69   Protection, 1993.

70   Fixings, 1993.

71 to 80 –

## Firecode

81   Firecode: fire precautions in new hospitals, 1987.

81   Supp 1, 1993.

82   Firecode: alarm and detection systems, 1989.

83   Fire safety in health care premises: general fire precautions*†

85   [Revision to Home Office draft guidance in preparation]

86   Firecode: assessing fire risks in existing hospital wards, 1987.

87   Firecode: textiles and furniture, 1993.

88   Fire safety in health care premises: guide to fire precautions in NHS housing in the community for mentally handicapped/ill people, 1986.

## New HTMs in preparation

Lifts

Combined heat and power

Telecommunications (telephone exchanges)

Washers for sterile production

Ventilation in healthcare premises

Risk management and quality assurance

Health Technical Memoranda published by HMSO can be purchased from HMSO bookshops in London (post orders to PO Box 276, SW8 5DT), Edinburgh, Belfast, Manchester, Birmingham and Bristol, or through good booksellers. HMSO provide a copy service for publications which are out of print; and a standing order service.

Enquiries about Health Technical Memoranda (but not orders) should be addressed to: NHS Estates, Department of Health, Marketing and Publications Unit, 1 Trevelyan Square, Boar Lane, Leeds LS1 6AE.

# About NHS Estates

NHS Estates is an Executive Agency of the Department of Health and is involved with all aspects of health estate management, development and maintenance. The Agency has a dynamic fund of knowledge which it has acquired during 30 years of working in the field. Using this knowledge NHS Estates has developed products which are unique in range and depth. These are described below.

NHS Estates also makes its experience available to the field through its consultancy services.

Enquiries should be addressed to: NHS Estates, Department of Health, 1 Trevelyan Square, Boar Lane, Leeds LS1 6AE. Tel: 0532 547000.

## Some other NHS Estates products

**Activity DataBase** – a computerised system for defining the activities which have to be accommodated in spaces within health buildings. *NHS Estates*

**Design Guides** – complementary to Health Building Notes, Design Guides provide advice for planners and designers about subjects not appropriate to the Health Building Notes series. *HMSO*

**Estatecode** – user manual for managing a health estate. Includes a recommended methodology for property appraisal and provides a basis for integration of the estate into corporate business planning. *HMSO*

**Capricode** – a framework for the efficient management of capital projects from inception to completion. *HMSO*

**Concode** – outlines proven methods of selecting contracts and commissioning consultants. Both parts reflect official policy on contract procedures. *HMSO*

**Works Information Management System** – a computerised information system for estate management tasks, enabling tangible assets to be put into the context of servicing requirements. *NHS Estates*

**Option Appraisal Guide** – advice during the early stages of evaluating a proposed capital building scheme. Supplementary guidance to Capricode. *HMSO*

**Health Building Notes** – advice for project teams procuring new buildings and adapting or extending existing buildings. *HMSO*

**Health Facilities Notes** – debate current and topical issues of concern across all areas of healthcare provision. *HMSO*

**Health Guidance Notes** – an occasional series of publications which respond to changes in Department of Health policy or reflect changing NHS operational management. Each deals with a specific topic and is complementary to a related Health Technical Memorandum. *HMSO*

**Encode** – shows how to plan and implement a policy of energy efficiency in a building. *HMSO*

**Firecode** – for policy, technical guidance and specialist aspects of fire precautions. *HMSO*

**Nucleus** – standardised briefing and planning system combining appropriate standards of clinical care and service with maximum economy in capital and running costs. *NHS Estates*

**Concise** – Software support for managing the capital programme. Compatible with Capricode. *NHS Estates*

Items noted "HMSO" can be purchased from HMSO Bookshops in London (post orders to PO Box 276, SW8 5DT), Edinburgh, Belfast, Manchester, Birmingham and Bristol or through good booksellers. Details of their standing order service are given at the front of this publication.

Enquiries about NHS Estates products should be addressed to: NHS Estates, Marketing and Publications Unit, Department of Health, 1 Trevelyan Square, Boar Lane, Leeds LS1 6AE.

## NHS Estates consultancy service

Designed to meet a range of needs from advice on the oversight of estates management functions to a much fuller collaboration for particularly innovative or exemplary projects.

Enquiries should be addressed to: NHS Estates Consultancy Service (address as above).

Printed in the United Kingdom for HMSO.
Dd.297565, C15, 12/93, 3396/4, 5673, 264323.